Blood Sugar Diet Solution

45 foods that help regulate blood sugar

By

Dr Chris Hollin Peters

Table of Contents

What should my glucose level be in my blood?

Which insulins are approved for diabetes treatment?

How do you take insulin? How many different ways can insulin be taken?

Which diabetes medications can be taken orally?

Chapter 3

Prevention

Are there additional diabetes treatment options?

Can diabetes type 1 be avoided?

Can diabetes's long-term complications be avoided?

Are prediabetes, type 2 diabetes, and gestational diabetes preventable conditions?

LIVING WITH When do I need to see my doctor?

Are foods high in sugar linked to diabetes?

OUTLOOK / PROGNOSIS What can I anticipate if I have been given a diabetes diagnosis?

How frequently should I visit my primary diabetes healthcare provider?

Is diabetes curable or reversible?

Introduction

Your body can't properly process and use the glucose in your food if you have diabetes. The problem of having too much glucose in your bloodstream is shared by all types of diabetes, each with its own unique set of causes. Insulin and/or medications are used as treatments. A healthy lifestyle can help prevent some types of diabetes.

Diabetes is a long-term condition that affects the body's ability to convert food into energy.

The majority of the food you eat is broken down by your body into sugar (glucose), which is then released into your bloodstream. Your pancreas releases insulin when your blood sugar goes up. Insulin let's blood sugar into your cells so that it can be used as energy.

Your body doesn't make enough insulin or doesn't use it as well as it should when you have diabetes. Too much sugar remains in your bloodstream when there isn't enough insulin or when your cells stop responding to insulin. That has the potential to result in serious health issues over time, including kidney disease, vision loss, and heart disease.

Diabetes doesn't have a cure yet, but losing weight, eating well, and exercising can really help.

Chapter 1
What is Diabetes?

Diabetes is a disease. When your body is unable to absorb sugar (glucose) into its cells and use it for energy, you develop diabetes. As a result, more sugar builds up in your bloodstream.

Diabetes management mistakes can have serious consequences, causing damage to your heart, kidneys, eyes, and nerves, among other organs and tissues.

Why do I have a high blood glucose level? What causes this to occur?

Breaking down food into its various nutrient sources is an important part of digestion. Your body converts carbohydrates like bread, rice, and pasta into sugar (glucose) when you eat them. When glucose enters your bloodstream, it needs assistance—a "key"—to get inside your body's cells, where it will be used. Cells are what make up your body's tissues and organs. Insulin is the help or "key" here.

Your pancreas, an organ behind your stomach, is responsible for the production of insulin, a hormone. Insulin is pumped into your bloodstream by your pancreas. Insulin is the "key" that opens the "door" in the cell wall, allowing glucose to enter your body's cells. The "fuel," or energy, that tissues and organs require to function properly is provided by glucose.

Those with diabetes:

Your pancreas does not produce enough insulin or any insulin at all.
Or, your pancreas produces insulin, but the cells in your body do not respond to it and are unable to use it as they normally would.
Glucose stays in your bloodstream and raises your blood glucose level if it cannot enter your cells.

How many different kinds of diabetes are there?

Types of diabetes include:

- *Diabetes mellitus*: An auto-immune disease is one in which your body attacks itself. Your pancreas' insulin-producing cells are destroyed in this scenario. Type 1 diabetes affects up to 10% of diabetes patients. It is typically diagnosed in young adults and children, but it can occur at any age. Previously, it was referred to as "juvenile" diabetes. Insulin needs to be taken every day by people who have Type 1 diabetes. It is also known as insulin-dependent diabetes as a result.

- ***Diabetes mellitus***: This type occurs when either your body doesn't produce enough insulin or your cells do not normally respond to the insulin. The most prevalent form of diabetes is this one. Type 2 diabetes affects up to 95% of diabetes patients. It usually happens to people who are middle-aged or older. Adult-onset diabetes and insulin-resistant diabetes are two additional terms used to describe Type 2. It might have been referred to by your grandparents or parents as "having a touch of sugar."

- **Prediabetes**: The stage that comes before Type 2 diabetes is this type. Although your blood glucose levels are higher than usual, they are not high enough to indicate Type 2 diabetes.
- **Diabetes at birth**: During pregnancy, some women develop this type. After giving birth, gestational diabetes typically disappears. However, you are more likely to develop Type 2 diabetes in later life if you have gestational diabetes.

Types of diabetes that are less common include:

- **Diabetes syndromes caused by genes**: Up to 4% of all cases of diabetes are accounted for by these uncommon inherited forms. Diabetes in infants and young people with maturity-onset diabetes are two examples.

- ***Diabetes caused by cystic fibrosis***: This is a type of diabetes that only those with this condition experience.
- ***Diabetes brought on by chemicals or drugs***: This happens after an organ transplant, after HIV/AIDS treatment, or when glucocorticoid steroid use is involved.

A distinct and uncommon condition known as diabetes insipidus causes your kidneys to produce a significant amount of urine.

How widespread is diabetes?

In the United States, approximately 1 in 10 people, or 34.2 million people of all ages, have diabetes. About 7.3 million adults aged 18 and older, or 1 in 5, are unaware that they have diabetes, or just under 3 percent of all adults in the United States. As people get older, more people are diagnosed with diabetes. Diabetes affects about one in four adults over the age of 65.

Who acquires diabetes? What are the potential dangers?

The factors that raise your risk vary depending on the kind of diabetes you end up getting.

The following are risk factors for type 1 diabetes:

- Having a parent or sibling with a history of Type 1 diabetes
- The pancreas has been damaged by something like an infection, a tumor, surgery, or an accident.
- Auto-antibodies (antibodies that erroneously attack your own tissues or organs) are present.
- Physical strain (such as an illness or surgery).
- Exposure to viruses that cause diseases.

The following are risk factors for prediabetes and type 2 diabetes:

Prediabetes or Type 2 diabetes in the family, whether it be a parent or a sibling.

- Being of Asian-American, Pacific Islander, Black, Hispanic, Native American, or other race
- Being overweight or obese.
- Having an elevated blood pressure
- Having high triglyceride levels and low HDL (the "good" cholesterol) levels.
- A lack of physical activity.
- Being older than 45.
- Having diabetes during pregnancy or giving birth to a child who weighs more than 9 pounds.
- Being affected by polycystic ovary syndrome.
- Having a history of stroke or heart disease.
- Having smoked.

The following are risk factors for gestational diabetes:

- Prediabetes or Type 2 diabetes in the family, whether it be a parent or a sibling.
- Being Asian-American, Native American, Hispanic, or African-American.
- Having been overweight or obese prior to becoming pregnant.
- Being older than 25 years old.

Chapter 2
SYMPTOMS AND CAUSES

What causes it?

Having an excess of glucose in your bloodstream is the root of all forms of diabetes. However, the reason for high blood glucose levels varies from diabetes type.

- *Diabetes type 1 is caused by*: This is a disease of the immune system. The cells in your pancreas that make insulin are attacked and destroyed by your body. If you don't have insulin, glucose builds up in your bloodstream and can't get into your cells. Some patients may also be affected by genes. Additionally, a virus may initiate an immune response.
- *Pre-diabetes and type 2 diabetes are brought on by:* The cells of your body

prevent insulin from functioning as it should to allow glucose into its cells. Insulin has become ineffective against the cells in your body. To overcome this resistance, your pancreas cannot keep up and produce sufficient insulin. The amount of glucose in your blood increases.

- ***Diabetes at birth:*** Your body's cells become more resistant to insulin as a result of hormones that are produced by the placenta during your pregnancy. To overcome this resistance, your pancreas is unable to produce sufficient insulin. Your bloodstream contains an excess amount of glucose.

What are diabetes's symptoms?
Diabetic symptoms include:

- Thirst increased.
- Sluggishness and fatigue.
- Vision that is hazy.

- Tingling or numbness in the hands or feet.
- Wounds that take a long time to heal
- Weight loss that wasn't planned.
- A lot of urination.
- Frequent infections with no explanation.
- Itchy mouth

Other symptoms in women include: Skin that is dry and scaly, as well as frequent infections with yeast or the urinary tract.

In men: diminished muscle strength, diminished sexual desire, and erectile dysfunction.

Signs of type 1 diabetes: Over the course of a few weeks or months, symptoms can manifest quickly. When you are a child, a teen, or a young adult, symptoms begin. Nausea, vomiting, stomach pains, and yeast infections or urinary tract infections are additional symptoms.

Symptoms of prediabetes and type 2 diabetes: Because they develop slowly over several years, you may not experience any symptoms at all or fail to notice them. Although pre-diabetes and type 2 diabetes are on the rise across all age groups, symptoms typically begin to manifest when you are an adult.

Diabetes at birth: Typically, you won't notice any symptoms. Between the 24th and 28th weeks of your pregnancy, you will be tested for gestational diabetes by your obstetrician.

What are diabetes's side effects?

Your body's tissues and organs can suffer serious damage if your blood glucose level stays high for an extended period of time. Over time, some complications can be fatal.

Problems include:

- Heart disease, chest pain, a heart attack, a stroke, high blood pressure, high cholesterol, and atherosclerosis are all examples of cardiovascular problems.

- Damage to the nerves (neuropathy), which results in numbness and tingling that starts in the toes or fingers and spreads.
- Nephropathy is damage to the kidney that can result in kidney failure, necessitate dialysis, or necessitate a transplant.
- A condition known as retinopathy that can cause blindness in the eyes; glaucoma and cataracts
- Damage to the feet, including damage to the nerves, insufficient blood flow, and poor wound and cut healing.
- Acne on the skin.
- Erection problems.
- loss of hearing
- Depression.
- Dementia.
- Issues with the teeth
- Diabetes gestational-related complications:

The mother: Pre-eclampsia (high blood pressure, excessive protein in the urine, swelling of the legs and feet), the possibility of gestational diabetes in subsequent pregnancies, and the possibility of developing diabetes in later life.

In the infant: Low blood sugar (hypoglycemia), a higher risk of developing Type 2 diabetes over time, and a death shortly after birth that is greater than normal.

Diagnosis and tests for diabetes, What tests are used to diagnose diabetes?

A blood test to measure your glucose level is used to diagnose and treat diabetes. Your blood glucose level can be measured using one of three tests: A1c test, random glucose test, and fasting glucose test.

- *Plasma glucose test during a fast*: After an eight-hour fast during which nothing but water was consumed, this test should be performed in the morning.

- ***Plasma glucose test at random***: This test does not require a rush and can be completed at any time.
- ***Test of A1C***: Your average blood glucose level over the past two to three months is provided by this test, which is also known as the HbA1C or glycated hemoglobin test. The amount of glucose attached to hemoglobin, the oxygen-carrying protein in your red blood cells, is measured by this test. Prior to this test, you do not need to sprint.
- ***Test for oral glucose tolerance***: After a night of fasting, the blood glucose level is first measured in this test. You then consume a sweet beverage. The glucose level in your blood is then checked at the first, second, and third hours.

Kind of test

Fasting

glucose test
Normal(mg/dL)
Under 100

Pre-diabetes(mg/dL)
100-125
Diabetes(mg/dL)
126 or higher
Irregular (whenever)
glucose test
Normal(mg/dL)
Under 140

Pre-diabetes(mg/dL)
140-199
Diabetes(mg/dL)
200 or higher
A1c test
Normal(mg/dL)
Under 5.7%

Pre-diabetes(mg/dL)
5.7 - 6.4%
Diabetes(mg/dL)

6.5% or higher
Oral glucose
resilience test
Normal(mg/dL)
Under 140
Pre-diabetes(mg/dL)
140-199
Diabetes(mg/dL)
200 or higher

- ***Gestational diabetes tests***: If you are pregnant, you will need to have two blood glucose tests. In a glucose challenge test, you drink a sugary beverage and have your glucose level checked after an hour. Prior to this test, you do not need to sprint. An oral glucose tolerance test will be performed (as previously mentioned) in the event that this test reveals a glucose level that is higher than normal (over 140 ml/dL).

- ***Diabetes mellitus***: Blood and urine samples will be taken and tested if your doctor suspects Type 1 diabetes. Auto-antibodies, which are a sign that your body is attacking itself, are examined in the blood. Ketones, which are a sign that your body is burning fat for energy, are checked for in the urine. Diabetes type 1 is indicated by these signs.

Who ought to have diabetes checked out?

You should get tested for diabetes if you have symptoms or risk factors. Diabetes can be managed more effectively and complications can be reduced or avoided earlier if it is discovered earlier. If a blood test shows that you have prediabetes, you and your doctor can work together to make changes to your lifestyle, like losing weight, exercising, and eating a healthy diet, to avoid or delay developing type 2 diabetes.

Additional recommendations for specific testing based on risk factors:

- *Diagnosis of type 1 diabetes:* Perform the test on children and young adults who have diabetes in their family. Alternate adults may also develop Type 1 diabetes, though less frequently. Therefore, it is essential to conduct testing on adults who present to the hospital and are found to have diabetes-related ketoacidosis. Ketoacidosis is a potentially fatal complication of Type 1 diabetes.
- *Diagnosis of type 2 diabetes*: Test adults over the age of 45, people between the ages of 19 and 44 who are overweight or obese and have one or more risk factors, pregnant women with type 2 diabetes, and children between the ages of 10 and 18 who are overweight or obese and have at least two risk factors.

- ***Diabetes at birth***: All pregnant women with diabetes diagnoses should be tested. All pregnant women should be tested between weeks 24 and 28. Your obstetrician may perform an earlier test on you if you have any other risk factors for gestational diabetes.

Diabetes Management and Treatment

How is diabetes managed?

Your entire body is affected by diabetes. You must control your risk factors in order to manage diabetes effectively, including:

Follow a diet plan

Take your prescribed medications

Get more exercise to keep your blood glucose levels as close to normal as possible.

Keep your HDL and LDL blood cholesterol and triglyceride levels as close to normal as you can.

Control your heart rate. Your BP shouldn't be higher than 140/90 mmHg.

You hold the keys to diabetes management by:

- Planning your meals and sticking to a healthy schedule are important. Eat vegetables, whole grains, beans, fruits, healthy fats, and little sugar on the Dash or Mediterranean diets. These diets are low in calories and fat but packed with nutrients and fiber. For assistance comprehending nutrition and meal planning, consult a registered dietitian.
- Regular exercise. Attempt to exercise for at least 30 minutes each day. Swim, walk, or do something you like.
- Gaining weight in a healthy way. Develop a weight loss strategy in collaboration with your healthcare team.
- Adhering strictly to instructions regarding the dosage and timing of insulin and other medications as prescribed.

- At home, keeping an eye on your blood pressure and glucose levels.
- Keeping your appointments with your healthcare providers and completing your doctor's orders for laboratory tests.
- Getting rid of your smoking habit

How do I measure the glucose level in my blood? Why is this crucial?

The results of a blood glucose test can help you make decisions about what to eat, how much you exercise, and any necessary medication or insulin adjustments or additions.

Using a blood glucose meter is the most common method for determining your blood glucose level. This test requires you to prick the side of your finger, apply a drop of blood to a test strip, and then insert the strip into the meter. The meter will then display your current glucose level. How frequently you'll need to check your glucose level will be explained to you by your doctor.

What is glucose monitoring on a continuous basis?

We now have yet another method for gauging glucose levels thanks to technological advancements. A tiny sensor that is inserted under your skin is used for continuous glucose monitoring. There is no need to poke your finger. Instead, the sensor can display your glucose levels at any time of day or night. Continuous glucose monitors may be an option for you if you ask your doctor about them.

What should my glucose level be in my blood?

Find out what your ideal blood glucose level should be from your healthcare team. They might have a particular range of targets for you. However, the majority of people attempt to maintain these goals for their blood glucose levels:

Before eating: between 80 and 130 mg/dL approximately two hours after eating: less than 180 mg/dL. If my blood glucose level is low, *what happens?*

Hypoglycemia is when blood glucose levels fall below the normal range (typically below 70 mg/dL). This is a signal from your body that you require sugar.

If you have hypoglycemia, you might experience the following symptoms:

- Shaking or weakness.
- Sweating and wet skin.
- A rapid heartbeat
- Dizziness.
- Hunger suddenly.
- Confusion.
- Skin is pale.
- Tongue or mouth numbness
- Irritability and anxiety
- Unsteadiness.

- Recurring nightmares and unrestful sleep
- Vision that is hazy.
- Seizures, headaches

If you don't control your hypoglycemia, you might pass out.

If my blood glucose level is high, what will happen?

Hyperglycemia is a condition in which your blood sugar levels are too high. A hyperglycemic state is:

A glucose level in the blood that is greater than 125 mg/dL when the person is fasting (no food or drink for at least eight hours). or a glucose level in the blood that is higher than 180 mg/dL within one to two hours of eating

How does diabetes get treated?

The type of diabetes you have, how well you manage your blood glucose levels, and any other health conditions you have are all factors in diabetes treatment.

1. *Diabetes mellitus*: You are required to take insulin every day if you have this type. Insulin is no longer produced by your pancreas.
2. *Diabetes mellitus*: Treatments for this type of diabetes can include insulin, medications (for both diabetes and conditions that are risk factors for diabetes), and changes to one's lifestyle, such as eating healthier foods, exercising more, and losing weight.
3. *Prediabetes*: The objective is to prevent you from developing diabetes if you have prediabetes. Treatments focus on risk factors that can be treated, like losing weight by exercising for at least 30 minutes five days a week and eating a healthy diet like the Mediterranean diet. As can be

seen in the prevention section of this research, many of the methods used to prevent diabetes are also used to treat it.

4. ***Diabetes at birth***: If you have this type and your glucose level isn't too high, changing your diet and getting regular exercise might be your first course of treatment. Your healthcare team may start you on insulin or medication if your glucose level is extremely high or the target goal is still not met.

Diabetes can be treated in one of the following ways with oral medications and insulin:

- Stimulates insulin production and release in your pancreas.
- Slows down the liver's release of glucose (the liver stores extra glucose).
- Blocks the breakdown of carbohydrates in your stomach or intestines, thereby making your tissues more insulin-responsive.

- Enables you to eliminate glucose from your body through increased urination.

Which diabetes medications can be taken orally?

The Food and Drug Administration has granted approval to over 40 diabetes medications. To discuss all of these drugs is beyond the scope of this research. Instead, we'll talk about the most common drug classes, how they work, and the names of a few drugs in each one. If you are a good candidate for medication, your healthcare team will decide. If that is the case, they will select the best diabetes medication.

The following drug classes treat diabetes:

- ***Sulfonylureas***: By increasing insulin production in the pancreas, these medications lower blood glucose levels. Glyburide (Micronase®, DiaBeta®), glimepiride (Amaryl®), and glipizide (Glucotrol®) are examples.

Glinides—also known as meglitinides—are By increasing insulin production in the pancreas, these medications lower blood glucose levels. Randin® 's repaglinide and Starlix®'s nateglinide are two examples.

- **Biguanides**: The liver produces less glucose as a result of these drugs. It also slows down the process by which carbohydrates become sugar and makes insulin work better in the body. An example is Metformin (Glucophage®).
- **Anti-alpha-glucosidase drugs**: By slowing down the breakdown of carbohydrates and reducing glucose absorption in the small intestine, these medications lower blood glucose levels. Precose®'s acarbose is one example.
- **Thiazolidinediones**: By allowing more glucose to enter muscles, fat, and the liver, these medications improve the way insulin works in the body. Pioglitazone (Actos®) and

rosiglitazone (Avandia®) are two examples.

- *GLP-1 analogs (additionally called incretin mimetics or glucagon-like peptide-1 receptor agonists):* These medications delay the stomach's emptying of food, reduce liver glucose release after meals, and increase insulin release. Byetta® exenatide, Victoza® liraglutide, Tanzeum® albiglutide, Rybelsus® semaglutide, and Trulicity® dulaglutide are all examples.

- *Dipeptidyl peptidase-4 inhibitors, also known as DPP-4 inhibitors*: These medications assist your pancreas in producing more insulin after meals. Additionally, they reduce the amount of glucose produced by the liver. Alogliptin (Nesina®), sitagliptin (Januvia®), saxagliptin (Onglyza®), and linagliptin (Tradjenta®) are, among others, examples.

- *Substances that block SGLT2, also known as sodium-glucose cotransporter 2 inhibitors*: Utilizing your kidneys, these medications enable you to eliminate glucose from your body through urine. Canagliflozin (Invokana®), dapagliflozin (Farxiga®), and empagliflozin (Jardiance®) are a few examples.
- *Sequestrants of bile acid*: Cholesterol and blood sugar levels are reduced by these drugs. Colestipol (Colestid®), cholestyramine (Questran®), and colesevelam (Welchol®) are all examples.
- *Agonist of dopamine*: The amount of glucose released by the liver is reduced by this medication. Bromocriptine (Cycloset®) is one example.

For optimal blood glucose management, many oral diabetes medications can be combined with insulin. Some of the above medications are available as a pill that combines two medications. Other medications, such as the

GLP-1 agonists semaglutide (Ozempic®) and lixisenatide (Adlyxin®), can be injected.

Always take your medication exactly as prescribed by your doctor. With them, discuss your specific inquiries and concerns.

Which insulins are approved for diabetes treatment?
Insulin for diabetes comes in many different varieties. If you require insulin, your healthcare team will discuss the various types and whether oral medications should be taken with it. A brief discussion of the various insulin types follows.

- *Insulins with a rapid action*: These insulins are taken 15 minutes before meals, peak at one hour (when they work best) and continue to work for two to four hours. Insulin aspart (NovoLog®), insulin lispro

(Humalog®), and insulin glulisine (Apidra®) are examples.

- ***Insulins that act quickly***: These insulins reach your bloodstream in about 30 minutes, peak in two to three hours, and last between three and six hours. Regular insulin (Humulin R®) is an example.

- ***Insulins with intermediate action***: These insulins work for up to 18 hours, peak in four to twelve hours, and reach your bloodstream in two to four hours.

- ***Insulin that lasts longer***: These insulins work to maintain steady blood sugar throughout the day. These insulins typically last about 18 hours. Insulins such as insulin detemir (Levemir®), insulin degludec (Tresiba®), and insulin glargine (Basaglar®, Lantus®, and Toujeo®) are examples.

Insulins that combine several different insulins exist. Xultophy®, Soliqua®, and other GLP-1 receptor agonist medications can also be used in conjunction with insulin.

How do you take insulin? How many different ways can insulin be taken?

Insulin is available in a variety of packaging options. Based on your preferences, lifestyle, insulin requirements, and insurance plan, you and your doctor will choose the best method of delivery. Here is a brief overview of the various options.

- *Syringe and needle*: You will use this technique to fill a needle with the appropriate amount of insulin after inserting it into an insulin vial and pulling back the syringe. The insulin will be injected into your buttocks, upper arm, or belly using a rotating needle. To maintain your desired blood glucose level, you may need to administer one or more shots daily.
- *Insulin stick*: This device has a cap that resembles a pen. They either come

with insulin cartridges that must be inserted and replaced after use or come prefilled with insulin.

- *Pump for Insulin*: Insulin pumps are small, computerized devices that you wear on your belt, in your pocket, or under your clothes. They are about the size of a small cell phone. Through a cannula, a small, flexible tube, they administer rapid-acting insulin all day, every day. Using a needle, the cannula is inserted beneath the skin. After that, the flexible tube beneath the skin is all that remains of the needle. The cannula should be changed every two to three days. A different kind of insulin pump doesn't use tubes and is attached to your skin directly.

- *An artificial pancreas, also known as an insulin delivery system with a closed loop, is:* An insulin pump is connected to a continuous glucose monitor in this system. Your blood glucose levels are checked every five minutes by the monitor, and the pump then administers the appropriate amount of insulin.

- *Inhaler of insulin:* By inserting an inhaler device into your mouth, inhalers enable you to inhale a powdered inhaler. The insulin is absorbed into your bloodstream after being inhaled into your lungs. Adults with Type 1 or Type 2 diabetes are the only people who are permitted to use inhalers.
- *Port for injecting insulin:* A short tube is inserted into the tissue beneath your skin in this method of delivery. A patch that sticks to the skin holds the port in place. You inject insulin through this port with an insulin pen or needle and syringe. Every few days, the port is changed. Instead of having to rotate injection sites, the port provides a single location.

- *Injector jet:* A fine spray of insulin is delivered through your skin using this needleless method and high pressure.

Are there additional diabetes treatment options?

Yes. A small number of people with Type 1 diabetes may be able to benefit from one of two types of transplants. Transplanting a pancreas is an option. However, in order to receive an organ transplant, you will need to deal with the side effects of immune-suppressing medications for the rest of your life. However, you may be able to stop taking insulin if the transplant is successful.

A pancreatic islet transplant is yet another type of transplant. In this procedure, an organ donor transplants clusters of islet cells—the cells that make insulin—into your pancreas to replace the ones that have been destroyed.

Immunotherapy is another treatment for Type 1 diabetes that is being studied. Immunotherapy has the potential to use medication to turn off the immune system components that cause Type 1 disease because Type 1 is an immune system disease.

Another treatment option that treats diabetes indirectly is bariatric surgery. If you have Type 2 diabetes, are considered to be obese (body mass index over 35), and are obese, bariatric surgery may be an option. People who have lost a lot of weight typically have much higher blood glucose levels.

Naturally, you will be prescribed additional medications to treat any existing health issues that increase your risk of developing diabetes. High cholesterol, high blood pressure, and other diseases related to the heart are examples of these conditions.

Chapter 3
PREVENTION

Are prediabetes, type 2 diabetes, and gestational diabetes preventable conditions?

Other diabetes risk factors, such as race and family history, cannot be changed, but you can manage some of them. In order to lower your risk of developing diabetes and improve these modifiable risk factors, adopt some of the healthy lifestyle habits listed below:

Follow a healthy diet, such as the Dash or Mediterranean diet. Keep a food diary and keep track of how many calories you eat. You can lose 12 pounds per week by cutting 250 calories per day.

Get your body moving. At least five days per week, aim for 30 minutes. Start slowly and work your way up to this amount, or divide these minutes into 10-minute segments that are easier to manage. Walking is a great way to work out.

Do your best to maintain a healthy weight. If you are pregnant, you should not lose weight, but you should talk to your obstetrician about healthy weight gain during your pregnancy.

Reduce your anxiety. Learn yoga, deep breathing exercises, relaxation techniques, and other useful strategies.

Reduce alcohol consumption. Men should limit their alcohol consumption to no more than two beverages per day; A single drink is the limit for women.

Get the recommended 7 to 9 hours of sleep each night.

Give up smoking.

Take the medications your doctor gives you to control your existing risk factors for heart disease (such as high cholesterol and blood pressure) or lower your risk of developing type 2 diabetes.

Consult your doctor if you think you may have prediabetes symptoms.

Can diabetes type 1 be avoided?

No. Diabetes type 1 is an auto-immune condition in which the body attacks itself. The reason why a person's body would attack itself is unknown to scientists. Genetic changes, for example, could also play a role.

Can diabetes's long-term complications be avoided?

The majority of diabetes-related illnesses and deaths are caused by chronic complications. Hyperglycemia (high blood sugar) typically lasts for several years before chronic complications occur. Patients with Type 2 diabetes may have signs of complications at the time of diagnosis due to the fact that these patients may have elevated blood sugar levels for several years before being diagnosed.

This research has already talked about diabetes complications. Although the complications can affect a variety of organ systems and range widely, many fundamental prevention principles are universal. These are some:

1. Follow your doctor's instructions for taking your insulin and/or insulin pills for diabetes.
2. Follow your doctor's orders and take all of your other medications to treat any risk factors, such as high cholesterol, high blood pressure, and other heart-related issues.
3. Keep an eye on your blood sugar levels.
4. Follow a diet that is good for you, like the Dash or Mediterranean diets. Avoid skipping meals.
5. At least 30 minutes of exercise every day, five days a week.
6. Keep your weight at a healthy level.
7. Be sure to drink plenty of water to stay hydrated.
8. If you smoke, give up.
9. To keep an eye on your diabetes and look for problems, see your doctor often.

OUTLOOK / PROGNOSIS What can I anticipate if I have been given a diabetes diagnosis?

Keeping your blood glucose level within the range that your doctor has recommended is the most important thing you can do if you have diabetes. These goals are, in general,:

Before eating: between 80 and 130 mg/dL approximately two hours after eating: less than 180 mg/dL. You will need to closely follow a treatment plan, which will likely include eating a custom diet, exercising for 30 minutes five times a week, quitting smoking, limiting alcohol consumption, and getting seven to nine hours of sleep each night. Always follow your doctor's instructions for taking your insulin and medications.

LIVING WITH When do I need to see my doctor?

If you have diabetes symptoms, you should see a doctor even if you haven't been diagnosed with it. If you have already been diagnosed with diabetes, you should talk to your doctor if your blood glucose levels are out of range, if your symptoms get worse, or if you start experiencing new symptoms.

Are foods high in sugar linked to diabetes?

Diabetes is not directly caused by sugar. Consuming foods with a lot of sugar can make you gain weight, which is a sign that you are more likely to get diabetes. The American Heart Association recommends no more than six teaspoons (25 grams) of sugar per day for women and nine teaspoons (36 grams) for men. Eating more sugar than this can cause a variety of health problems as well as weight gain.

All of these negative health effects have been linked to diabetes development or can make complications worse.

Gaining weight can,

Raise cholesterol, triglyceride, and blood pressure levels.

Increase your danger of heart disease.

Cause liver fat to build up.

Result in tooth decay.

What kind of medical professionals might be a part of my diabetes care team?

The majority of diabetics see their primary care physician first. An endocrinologist or pediatric endocrinologist, a doctor who treats diabetes patients, might be able to help you. An ophthalmologist (an eye doctor), a nephrologist (a kidney doctor), a cardiologist (a heart doctor), a podiatrist (a foot doctor), a neurologist (a doctor of the nerves and brain), a gastroenterologist (a doctor of the digestive tract), a registered dietician, nurse practitioners/physician assistants, a diabetes educator, a pharmacist, a personal trainer, a social worker.

How frequently should I visit my primary diabetes healthcare provider?

If you are receiving insulin injections, you should visit your doctor at least once every three to four months. You should see your doctor at least once every four to six months if you manage your diabetes through diet or medication. If your blood sugar isn't being controlled or your diabetes complications are getting worse, you might need to come in more often.

Is diabetes curable or reversible?

The responses to these questions are not as straightforward as they appear. Reversing diabetes may or may not be possible, depending on the type of diabetes and the specific cause. The more common term for successfully reversing diabetes is "remission."

Diabetes type 1 is a disease of the immune system with a genetic component. Traditional treatments cannot reverse this type of diabetes. To survive, you need insulin for life. The most advanced method of keeping glucose within a narrow range at all times and most closely mimicking the body is providing insulin through an artificial pancreas (insulin pump, continuous glucose monitor, and computer program). A pancreas transplant or pancreas islet transplant is the closest thing to a Type 1 cure. To be eligible, transplant candidates must meet stringent requirements. It's not for everyone, and it means having to deal with the side effects of immunosuppressant medications and taking them for life.

With a lot of effort and motivation, prediabetes and type 2 diabetes can be reversed. All of your disease risk factors would need to be changed. This requires regular exercise, healthy eating, and weight loss (such as a plant-based, low-carb, low-sugar, healthy fat diet, for example). Your blood pressure and cholesterol levels should also fall within the normal range as a result of these efforts. It has been demonstrated that some individuals with Type 2 diabetes can enter remission following bariatric surgery, which reduces the size of the stomach. This is a significant operation that comes with its own risks and problems.

When you have gestational diabetes, your condition lasts until your child is born. Having gestational diabetes, on the other hand, is a risk factor for Type 2 diabetes.

The good news is that diabetes can be controlled successfully. Talking to your doctor about how well you can manage your Type 1 or Type 2 diabetes is a good idea.

Is diabetes a killer?

Yes, diabetes can have devastating effects on your body if it is left untreated and undiagnosed (severely high or low glucose levels). Diabetes can result in a coma, heart attack, stroke, kidney failure, and heart failure. Your death may result from these complications. Adults with diabetes are particularly vulnerable to cardiovascular disease, which is the leading cause of death.

What effects does COVID-19 have on diabetics?

Even though having diabetes might not necessarily make you more likely to get COVID-19, if you do get the virus, you are more likely to get more serious problems. As your body fights off the infection if you get COVID-19, your blood sugar levels are likely to rise. Immediately notify your healthcare team if you contract COVID-19.

What effects does diabetes have on your kidneys, nerves, eyes, feet, and heart?

The tissues and organs of our body are lined with blood vessels. They surround the cells of our body and transport oxygen, nutrients, and other substances through blood as a means of exchange. Diabetes, to put it simply, prevents glucose, the body's fuel, from entering cells and damages blood vessels near or in these organs and those that nourish nerves. Organs, nerves, and tissues may begin to fail if they are unable to obtain the necessary nutrients. "Proper function" refers to the blood vessels in your heart, such as the arteries, not being damaged (narrowed or blocked). This means that waste products can be removed from your blood by your kidneys. This indicates that the blood vessels in your retina, the part of your eye that gives you vision, remain intact in your eyes. This indicates that blood is flowing to your feet and that your nerves are being fed. Damage caused by diabetes prevents normal function.

What causes diabetes to result in amputation?

Diabetes that is not managed can result in poor circulation. You are more likely to get cuts and sores that can lead to infections that won't heal completely if you don't have access to oxygen and nutrients (which are carried by blood). Poor blood flow is more likely to affect the parts of your body that are farthest away from your heart, which pumps blood. Therefore, if an infection develops and healing is poor, you may need to have parts of your body, such as your toes, feet, legs, and fingers, amputated.

Is diabetes a factor in blindness?

Yes. Diabetes that is not controlled can cause damage to the blood vessels in the retina, which can result in blindness. See an ophthalmologist or primary care physician as soon as possible if you are experiencing changes in your vision but have not yet been diagnosed with diabetes.

Is hearing loss possible with diabetes?

Although researchers do not yet have definitive answers, diabetes and hearing loss appear to be linked. A recent study found that people with diabetes had twice as much hearing loss as people without diabetes, Additionally, prediabetes patients had a 30% higher rate of hearing loss than those with normal blood glucose levels. Researchers believe that diabetes damages the inner ear blood vessels, but more research is required.

Can diabetes cause dizziness or headaches?

If your blood glucose level is too low, usually below 70 mg/dL, you may experience headaches or dizziness. This is called hypoglycemia. You can learn about the other symptoms that hypoglycemia causes. Hypoglycemia is common in Type 1 diabetics and can occur in some Type 2 diabetics who take insulin (insulin moves glucose from the blood into your cells) or sulfonylurea medications.

Is hair loss possible with diabetes?

Diabetes can, in fact, lead to hair loss. Diabetes that is not managed can result in persistently high blood glucose levels. As a result, hair follicles and damaged blood vessels prevent oxygen and nutrients from reaching the cells that require them. Hair growth can be affected by changes in hormone levels brought on by stress. Your immune system attacks itself in Type 1 diabetes, which can also lead to a condition known as alopecia areata, which causes hair loss.

Which kinds of diabetes call for insulin?

Insulin is necessary for life for people with Type 1 diabetes. Your body has attacked your pancreas and destroyed the cells that make insulin if you have Type 1 diabetes. Your pancreas produces insulin, but it doesn't work properly if you have Type 2 diabetes. Insulin may be required to transport glucose from the bloodstream to the cells of the body where it is needed for energy in some people with Type 2 diabetes. If you have gestational diabetes, you might or might not need to take insulin. Your healthcare provider will check your blood glucose level, look at other risk factors, and decide on a treatment plan in the event that you are pregnant or have Type 2 diabetes. This plan may include a combination of lifestyle changes, insulin taken orally, and other medications. Your treatment plan is unique, just like you are.

Can diabetes occur at birth? Is it inherited?

Diabetes does not occur naturally; however, Type 1 diabetes typically begins in childhood. Diabetes and pre-hypertension both progress slowly over time. Diabetes gestation is common during pregnancy. Genetics, according to researchers, may play a role or contribute to Type 1 diabetes development. It could be caused by a virus or something in the environment. You are more likely to develop Type 1 diabetes if you have a family history of the disease. You are more likely to develop prediabetes, type 2 diabetes, or gestational diabetes if you have a family history of either of those conditions.

What exactly is diabetic ketoacidosis?

Ketoacidosis caused by diabetes is a life-threatening condition. It occurs when glucose is not being used as an energy source and your liver breaks down fat to use as energy due to a lack of insulin. The liver breaks down fat into ketones, which are used as fuel. If you haven't eaten in a long time and your body needs fuel, ketones will naturally form and be used. When fat is broken down too quickly for the body to process, ketones form and accumulate in the blood. Ketoacidosis is a condition in which your blood becomes acidic as a result. Uncontrolled Type 1 diabetes and, less frequently, Type 2 diabetes can both lead to diabetes-related ketoacidosis. A basic metabolic panel and the presence of ketones in your urine or blood are used to diagnose diabetes-related ketoacidosis. The condition can lead to a coma or even death over the course of several hours.

What exactly is HHNS, short for hyperglycemic hyperosmolar nonketotic syndrome?

Compared to diabetes-related ketoacidosis, hyperglycemic hyperosmolar nonketotic syndrome (HHNS) develops more slowly over days to weeks. It usually happens when people with Type 2 diabetes are sick or stressed, especially the elderly. HHNS is characterized by frequent urination, drowsiness, lack of energy, and dehydration as well as a blood glucose level greater than 600 mg/dL. Ketones in the blood have nothing to do with HHNS. It may result in a coma or death. You will require hospital treatment.

If I have protein in my urine, what does this indicate?

This indicates that your kidneys are allowing protein to pass through and now produce urine. Proteinuria is the term for this condition. A sign of kidney damage is the continued presence of protein in your urine.

The fundamentals of glucose control

Carbohydrates like cereal, pasta, fruits, milk, dessert, and bread are typically to blame for elevated blood sugar levels. A meal plan is very important for diabetics because it tells them what foods to eat. It ought to be sufficient to accommodate your eating habits and schedule. Include the following in a good meal plan:

Glycemic index Carb counting Plate method Foods with low glycemic index values are better than foods with high glycemic index values for stabilizing blood sugar. The physiological ability of dietary carbohydrates to lower or raise the level of blood sugar in relation to the type of food consumed by a diabetic patient is the primary factor that determines the glycemic index. Foods with a relatively high glycemic index have ratings above 50 and typically fall between 75 and 100. The glycemic index values of foods that you can include in your Diabetes Diet Plan can be found on the Glycemic Index Food Chart.

Chapter 4
45 foods that help regulate blood sugar

A good meal plan helps you stay on track with your weight, lowers your cholesterol, lowers your blood sugar, and lowers your blood pressure. Diabetes type 2 can be reduced with a healthy diet and regular exercise to stay at a healthy weight. You can check out diabetic-friendly, delicious recipes that will help you lower your blood sugar levels without sacrificing flavor or variety!

45 foods that can help you maintain or lower your blood sugar are on this list:

1. Beans
2. Spinach
3. Collard green

4. Mustard greens

5. Sweet potatoes

6. Berries

7. Tomatoes

8. Oatmeal

9. Nuts

10. Mushrooms

11. Cauliflower

12. Cherries

13. Coconut

14. Apple

15. Peaches

16. Whole wheat bread

17. Carrots

18. Broccoli

19. Peas

20. Milk

21. Yogurt

22. Lentils

23. Grapes

24. Pears

25. Brown rice

26. Peanuts

27. Hummus

28. Cashews
29. Green beans
30. Oranges
31. Plums and prunes
32. Fish
33. Cinnamon
34. Garlic
35. Healthy fats
36. Chia seeds
37. Chili peppers
38. Vinegar
39. Lean meats
40. Figs
41. Dates
42. Barley
43. Pasta
44. Quinoa
45. Apricots

1. Beans

Beans are full of fiber and help you feel fuller for longer. Black beans, like all beans, have some carbohydrates, but they also have a lot of dietary fiber, protein, and other nutrients, which helps them have a low glycemic index. As a result, the Diabetes Food Chart gives them a prominent spot.

2. Spinach

Spinach is a vegetable that can be eaten all year round and is a good source of vitamins, folate, chlorophyll, manganese, calcium, potassium, zinc, phosphorus, protein, carotene, and other nutrients. It also contains manganese. Because it has a glycemic index close to zero, spinach helps diabetic patients maintain stable blood glucose levels.

3. Collard greens

Collard greens are cruciferous vegetables and include the following: kale, rutabaga, Brussels sprouts, cabbage, turnips, and other vegetables They are known to stabilize lipids, insulin, and blood glucose levels in type 2 diabetics, provide a lot of nutrients at low calories, and they lower blood glucose levels in patients with type 1 diabetes.

4. Mustard greens

Leaf-mustard greens are very low in calories and fat (27 calories per 100 grams of raw leaves). However, its dark-green leaves are loaded with vitamins, minerals, and phytonutrients. It also has a lot of dietary fiber, which prevents cholesterol from being absorbed in the gut and helps control cholesterol levels.

5. Sweet potatoes

Boiling sweet potatoes, which are the healthiest member of the potato family and have a glycemic index of 44, are regarded as a superfood for diabetics. Even if you have diabetes, eating sweet potatoes in moderation will help you maintain healthy blood sugar levels.

6. Berries

Fructose, a natural sugar found in berries, does not need to be metabolized; Consequently, the body tolerates the fruit well. Take two servings, but always check to see what works best for you.

7. Tomatoes

When consumed in moderation, fresh tomatoes are not a problem for controlling blood sugar levels. For instance, one medium whole tomato has 4.8 g of carbohydrates and 1.5 g of fiber, or the equivalent of 3.3 g of net carbs, while one cup of cherry tomatoes contains 5.8 g of carbohydrates and 1.8 g of fiber, which is the same as 4 g of net carbs. It has an estimated glycemic index between 2 and 4.

8. Oatmeal

Studies have demonstrated that consuming foods high in fiber and whole grains reduces diabetes risk by nearly 35 to 42%. Whole grains and a lot of fiber make up oatmeal. It also has soluble fiber, which slows down the rate of glucose absorption in the GIT and keeps blood sugar levels in the right range.

9. Nuts

According to research, consuming nuts on a daily basis may assist in controlling type 2 diabetes. It is essential to keep in mind that nuts have a glycemic index of 14 to 21—a significantly lower number. In comparison to the most popular snacks that most people eat, like crackers, they have relatively few carbohydrates.

10. Mushrooms

Although the glycemic index is always considered to be low, it can fluctuate depending on the kind of mushroom you choose. In addition to providing a novel flavor to a meal, it offers a unique set of nutritional benefits. Due to their nutritional value and beefy texture, portabella mushrooms are utilized as a meat substitute. There are 22 calories per 100 grams.

11. Cauliflower

In terms of glycemic load, cruciferous vegetables like cauliflower are extremely beneficial. Due to their anti-cancer and heart disease properties, these vegetables frequently appear in health news. This one-of-a-kind blend of phytonutrients is very healthy and well absorbed by the body when taken on a regular basis. This type of vegetable can be rotated so that you don't eat the same one every day.

12. Cherries

The glycemic index of these fruits is relatively low. Even though it isn't as low as some vegetables, it is thought to be good for diabetics. When creating a list of foods with a low glycemic index, it is unquestionably a fruit to take into consideration.

13. Coconut

Coconut has a lot of saturated fat, but if you use it sparingly, it won't affect your blood glucose levels too much. Coconuts add flavor to many different dishes. Coconut water, coconut milk, coconut flour, its flesh, and other parts can be used. However, in order to determine the glycemic index and the nutritional benefits, it is essential to know which component you are using.

14. An apple

This is due to the fact that apples have a low glycemic index of 39 and provide a wide range of nutritional benefits, including fiber, vitamins, and minerals. It doesn't need much preparation, doesn't need any special storage, and is also easy to carry.

15. Peaches

Peaches are an excellent seasonal food to store. They have a natural sweetness that you can enjoy, and when eaten in moderation, they can control blood sugar levels. Even though the GI changes when peaches are used in a dessert, fresh peaches shouldn't cause any problems. It has a GI rank of 28.

16. Whole wheat bread

In recent years, whole wheat bread has become increasingly popular. This is because white bread is thought to be bad for you. Wheat bread, on the other hand, has a GI of 49. This is due to the fact that it is processed differently than white bread, resulting in greater nutritional benefits.

17. Carrots

Carrot beta carotene, which is high in vitamin A and helps with vision, can be combined with peas to make a delicious meal that has a low glycemic index. The glycemic index of carrots is 19.

18. Broccoli

Broccoli is a superfood that appears on nearly every list of healthy foods. They are well-known for their high nutritional value, fiber, minerals, and vitamins. On the GI scale, they have a very low value of 10, so the body can handle them very well.

19. Peas

100 grams of these peas have 81 calories each. Additionally, they contain a fair amount of potassium and a lot of fiber. Additionally, it provides protein and vitamin C. 39 is its glycemic index.

20. Milk

Is well-known for its high protein content, calcium, and vitamin D content. Because milk is one of the foods with a glycemic index of 31 and falls under the category of low GI foods, it is perfectly acceptable for diabetics to drink milk.

21. Yogurt

Yogurt is well-known for its active and live cultures, which provide beneficial bacteria that aid in digestion. Yogurt, whether unsweetened or sweetened with artificial sugars, is still one of the low-GI foods. On the other hand, low-fat yogurt is suggested. It has a 33 glycemic index. Additionally, it's a good idea to eat yogurt without any artificial flavors or sweeteners.

22. Lentils

Lentils contain a lot of vitamins, minerals, and fiber. When it comes to a blood sugar-conscious diet, they are frequently overlooked and are slowly gaining popularity. They have a Glycemic Index of 30.

23. Grapes

Grapes are extremely sweet, and many diabetic dieters mistakenly believe they should be avoided when dieting. Grapes, whether white or red, can be enjoyed in a variety of ways. The glycemic index, which ranges from 43 to 53 depending on the variety, is considered low.

24. Pears

Pears are frequently compared to apples, but their nutritional content and flavor are distinct. If you're looking for a food with a low glycemic index, they're a great option. They have a glycemic index of 41.

25. Brown rice

The majority of diabetics consume brown rice frequently. This is due to the fact that a serving of brown rice has a glycemic rank of 55, whereas a serving of white rice has a glycemic rank of 87.

26. Peanuts

Peanuts can be consumed as a snack, alongside butter, or even with sauce. They are very effective at keeping someone alert and are considered legumes. Additionally, they excel at maintaining blood sugar levels. Their rank on the glycemic index is 6.

27. Hummus
Chickpea-based Hummus ranks lower. This is because they also contain lemons, olive oil, and tahini. Although their GI is almost zero, portion control is still necessary to avoid discomfort in the gastrointestinal tract. Six is the glycemic index.

28. Cashews
These healthy nuts can be consumed whenever you like. Both polyunsaturated and monounsaturated fats benefit from them. Additionally, it is a great source of iron and magnesium. If you buy organic cashew nut butter, it is also good for you. They have a GI of only 2.

29. Green Beans

Green Beans in a can are one of the most common foods that are served as a side dish. They are an excellent source of fiber, vitamin C, and minerals in addition to being relatively low on the GI scale. They supply antioxidants that aid in the fight against free radicals and prevent inflammation, both of which help to strengthen the immune system. They have a 15 glycemic index.

30. Oranges

Oranges are a great fruit to eat in the early stages of a cold to boost your immune system because of their high vitamin C content. They can be used as a fruit in the morning, in a smoothie, or as a constant boost. It has a 40 glycemic index.

31. Plums and Prunes

Plums and prunes are regarded as low-glycemic foods. Although their sizes may vary, they contain a significant amount of nutrition. Plums and prunes have glycemic indexes of 24 and 29, respectively.

32. Fish

Fish is good for diabetics because it is a good source of low proteins. They are known to be high in omega 3, a type of fat that protects against diabetes and strengthens the heart. Blood sugar levels can be significantly reduced by including seafood in your diet and eating at least two or more servings per week.

33. Cinnamon

Though many of us sprinkle cinnamon on our morning drinks, you might be surprised to learn that this wonderful spice has many positive effects on our health. Cinnamon has been shown to lower blood sugar levels, in addition to lowering bad cholesterol and increasing good cholesterol.

34. Garlic

Many people are afraid of garlic because it causes bad breath. However, it is known that garlic extract raises insulin levels for diabetics. As a result, it has been shown to lower blood sugar levels.

35. Healthy fats

Avocados, nuts, olive oil, salmon, tuna, and trout are all examples of foods that contain healthy fats. Monounsaturated fats found in all of them aid in lowering insulin resistance.

36. Chia seeds

Chia seeds are tiny, dark seeds that have a nutty flavor. Healthy fats, vitamins, fiber, and antioxidants abound in abundance in them. According to one of the studies," Chia seeds help raise blood sugar levels. Additionally, it lowers the risk of heart disease in type-2 diabetics.

37. Chili Peppers

Capsicum chili peppers have been grown for thousands of years and have been used for food, medicine, and decoration. The ability of chili peppers to activate the vanillin transient receptor is what makes them effective as medicines. Anxiety, neuropathic and inflammatory pain, and the way our bodies process fats are all linked to this receptor. Additionally, it is a crucial insulin regulator. Extracts aimed at pharmacological strategies for diabetes treatment have been produced as a result of this study.

38. Vinegar

Vinegar has been used for centuries to treat a wide range of health issues, such as controlling blood sugar, dandruff, excessive sweating, fungal infections, and even heartburn. Two tablespoons of ACV at bedtime helped patients with type II diabetes control their fasting blood glucose levels, according to a study that was published in Diabetes Care.

39. Lean meats

Protein-rich foods and lean meats are essential components of any diet. They consist of: meats, fish, chicken, cheese, and products made from soy Protein and fat content make these items distinct from one another.

40. Figs

Despite the fact that dried figs are available year-round, nothing beats the unique texture and flavor of fresh figs for reviving taste. It has long been known that the fig leaves have anti-diabetic properties and can lower the amount of insulin required by diabetics.

41. Dates

Dates often get a bad rap, as do peanuts and honey, two healthy but relatively dangerous foods for diabetes. However, these foods can help lower LDL (bad) cholesterol. Particularly for diabetics, portion control with these foods becomes crucial.

42. Barley

Barley 14 grams of fiber are contained in a cup of cooked whole-grain barley. 11g of the fiber is insoluble and 3g soluble. 6 grams of fiber—2 grams soluble and 4 grams insoluble—can be found in one cup of cooked pearl barley. When diabetics consume foods high in carbohydrates, their blood glucose levels change. The glycemic index of barley is 25.

43. Pasta

Pasta, in contrast to potatoes and white bread, has a relatively low glycemic impact. Because of its infamously high carbohydrate content, pasta is feared by many diabetics. However, pasta can be safely consumed on a diabetic diet if the proportions are right. To keep blood sugars low, choose whole grain pasta with a lot of fiber and small serving sizes.

44. Quinoa

Quinoa is a great way to keep your blood sugar in check. Protein, fiber, vitamins, minerals, phytochemicals, and a low glycemic index make up the bulk of whole grain, which helps maintain even blood sugar levels. Quinoa can be incorporated into a diabetic diet in a variety of ways because it is flavorful and easy to cook.

45. Apricots

Apricots have a delicate flavor and are sweet. They are worth including in a diabetic diet because they contain a wide range of nutrients.

Due to their low glycemic index, apricots can satisfy your sweet tooth without affecting your blood sugar levels. When consumed in small quantities, dried apricots are also an excellent alternative.

Chapter 5
14 Simple Ways to Lower Your Blood Sugar

Managing prediabetes or diabetes requires knowing how to naturally lower your blood sugar levels. Think about doing things like working out more often, getting more fiber in your diet, including more snacks, and getting more probiotics in your diet.

Diabetes and prediabetes are both associated with high blood sugar, or hyperglycemia. When your blood sugar is high but not high enough to be considered diabetes, you have prediabetes.

Most of the time, your body uses insulin, a hormone that lets your cells use the sugar in your blood that is circulating in your body, to control your blood sugar levels. As a result, insulin is the most significant factor in controlling blood sugar levels.

However, hyperglycemia can be caused by a number of factors that make it difficult to control blood sugar.

When the liver produces too much glucose, the body makes too little insulin, or the body can't use insulin properly, these are all internal causes of high blood sugar. Insulin resistance is the latter state.

Dietary choices, certain medications, a sedentary lifestyle, and stress are all external factors.

According to researchers, 13% of adults in the United States have diabetes, and another 34.5% have prediabetes. This indicates that nearly half of all adults in the United States have diabetes or prediabetes.

Because chronically high blood sugar levels can result in complications that can be life-threatening or endanger a person's limbs, blood sugar management is especially important for diabetics.

You can naturally lower your blood sugar levels in **14 easy, evidence-based ways**

1.Exercise
Regular exercise can improve insulin sensitivity and assist you in achieving and maintaining a moderate weight.
Your cells are able to use the sugar in your bloodstream more efficiently if they are insulin-sensitive.
Additionally, exercise assists your muscles in utilizing blood sugar for energy and contraction.

If you have trouble controlling your blood sugar, you might want to check your levels every time you exercise and before bed. This will help you understand how you react to various activities and maintain stable blood sugar levels.
In addition, the practice of so-called "exercise snacks" has been suggested by researchers as a

means of lowering blood sugar and preventing the harm that can result from sitting all day.

Breaking up your sitting time every 30 minutes for a few minutes throughout the day with exercise snacks is all that is required. Light walking and simple resistance exercises like squats and leg raises are among the suggested exercises.

Weightlifting, brisk walking, running, biking, dancing, hiking, swimming, and other useful forms of exercise are also available. In fact, a sedentary lifestyle is preferable to any activity that regularly gets you moving, regardless of its intensity.

In addition, keep in mind that even if you find it difficult to exercise for extended periods of time throughout the week, doing so in shorter sessions can still provide you with numerous advantages. For instance, try exercising for 10 minutes three times per day for five days, aiming for 150 minutes per week.

2. Control your carb intake

Your blood sugar levels are strongly influenced by your carb intake.

The body converts carbohydrates into sugars, primarily glucose. The body then uses and stores insulin for energy.

This process fails, and blood glucose levels can rise if you consume an excessive amount of carbohydrates or have issues with insulin function.

As a result, the American Diabetes Association (ADA) advises diabetics to track their carbohydrate intake and keep track of how many they need.

According to some studies, this can assist you in making appropriate meal plans, further enhancing blood sugar management.

Additionally, numerous studies demonstrate that a low-carb diet aids in lowering blood sugar levels and preventing spikes in blood sugar.

It is essential to keep in mind that no-carb and low-carb diets are not the same thing.

While keeping an eye on your blood sugar, you can still consume some carbohydrates. Whole grains, on the other hand, have a higher nutritional value and contribute to a reduction in blood sugar levels when eaten in preference to processed grains and refined carbs.

3. Consume more fiber

It slows the digestion of carbohydrates and the absorption of sugar, resulting in a more gradual rise in blood sugar levels.
Fiber can be classified as either soluble or insoluble.
While both are important, it has been demonstrated that soluble fiber improves blood sugar management, whereas insoluble fiber does not.
Your body's ability to control blood sugar can be improved and blood sugar lows can be reduced by eating a diet high in fiber. You might be able to better manage type 1 diabetes with this.

The following foods are high in fiber:

Whole grains, vegetables, legumes, and the recommended daily intake of fiber for men and women is approximately 35 grams. That amounts to approximately 14 grams per 1,000 calories.

4. Water

Drink plenty of water to stay hydrated. Drinking enough water can help you maintain healthy blood sugar levels.
It helps your kidneys eliminate any excess sugar through urine, preventing dehydration.

According to one review of observational studies, people who consumed more water had a lower risk of developing high blood sugar levels. Drinking water on a regular basis may rehydrate the body, lower blood sugar levels, and lower the risk of developing diabetes.

Keep in mind that the best drinks are water and other drinks without calories. Sugar-sweetened foods should be avoided because they can raise blood glucose levels, cause weight gain, and raise the risk of developing diabetes.

5. Use portion control

How many calories you consume and keep a moderate weight.

As a result, it has been demonstrated that controlling one's weight lowers the risk of developing type 2 diabetes and helps maintain healthy blood sugar levels.

Additionally, portion control prevents spikes in blood sugar, Some helpful hints for controlling portion sizes are as follows:

Keep a food journal, eat slowly, and weigh your portions. Avoid all-you-can-eat restaurants. Read food labels and check the serving sizes.

6. Choose foods with a low glycemic index (GI).

The glycemic index (GI) measures how quickly your body absorbs and breaks down carbohydrates. Your blood sugar levels will rise more quickly as a result of this.

On a scale from 0 to 100, the GI classifies foods as low, medium, and high. Foods with a GI of 55 or lower are considered low-GI.

How a food affects your blood sugar levels is determined by the amount and type of carbohydrates you consume. Consuming foods with a low glycemic index (GI) has been shown to lower blood sugar levels in diabetics.

Foods with a GI range from low to moderate include:

Bulgur barley, unsweetened Greek yogurt, oats, beans, lentils, legumes, whole wheat pasta, and vegetables that aren't starchy are all good sources of protein and healthy fats.

7. Stress

Try to control how much stress you have. Stress can affect how much sugar is in your blood.

Your body releases hormones called glucagon and cortisol when you're stressed, which raise blood sugar levels.

Exercise, deep relaxation, and meditation were found to significantly reduce stress and blood sugar levels in a student study.

Yoga and mindfulness-based stress reduction may also help people with chronic diabetes improve their insulin secretion.

8. Glucose level

You can better manage your blood sugar levels by monitoring your glucose levels.

Using a glucometer, a portable blood glucose meter, you can do this at home. You can talk to your doctor about this option.

You can determine whether your medications or meals need to be altered by keeping track. Additionally, it helps you understand how certain foods affect your body.

Try measuring your levels on a daily basis and recording the results in a log. Additionally, it might be more beneficial to track your blood sugar in pairs, such as before and after exercise or two hours after a meal.

If a meal spikes your blood sugar, this can show you whether you need to make minor adjustments rather than completely avoiding your favorite foods. Alterations include substituting non-starchy vegetables for a starchy side or limiting them to a handful.

9. Get enough good sleep

Getting enough sleep is good for your health and good for your mood.

In point of fact, poor sleeping patterns and a lack of rest can have an effect on insulin sensitivity and blood sugar levels, raising the risk of developing type 2 diabetes. They can also make people hungry and make them gain weight.

In addition, lack of sleep raises levels of the hormone cortisol, which, as previously mentioned, is crucial to controlling blood sugar levels.

Quality and quantity of sleep are two aspects of adequate sleep. Adults should get at least 7–8 hours of good sleep each night,

Try to improve your sleep quality by:

Create a bedtime routine and avoid working in your bedroom by taking a warm bath or shower before bed. Try meditation or guided imagery. Avoid alcohol and caffeine late in the day. Get regular exercise. Limit screen time before bed. Keep your bedroom cool. Use calming scents like lavender. Consume foods that are high in magnesium and chromium. Micronutrient deficiencies have been linked to diabetes and high blood sugar levels. Chromium and magnesium deficiency are two such examples.

10. Carbohydrate and fat metabolism are influenced by chromium.

It may increase insulin's effectiveness, assisting in the regulation of blood sugar

Foods high in chromium include:

Meats, whole grain products, fruits, vegetables, and nuts. However, the underlying mechanisms of this proposed connection are not completely understood, and research has produced conflicting results. Therefore, additional research is required. It has also been demonstrated that magnesium raises blood sugar levels. In point of fact, a diet high in magnesium is linked to a significantly lower risk of developing diabetes.

Conversely, diabetes sufferers may experience insulin resistance and impaired glucose tolerance if they have low magnesium levels.

However, taking magnesium supplements probably won't help you if you already consume a lot of magnesium-rich foods and have adequate blood magnesium levels.

Foods high in magnesium include:

Whole grains, dark chocolate, avocado, beans, dark leafy greens, squash, and pumpkin seeds, tuna, and You might want to think about including particular foods in your diet. Numerous plants and foods are known to have medicinal properties.

11. Consider adding specific foods to your diet However, a lack of human studies or small sample sizes contribute to the low quality of the evidence on these ingredients. As a result, no definitive recommendations regarding their application can be made.

The following foods may help prevent diabetes:

VINEGAR from apple cider. This ingredient may delay stomach emptying after a meal, which may reduce blood sugar levels, according to earlier research.
CINNAMON. By slowing the digestion of carbohydrates and increasing insulin sensitivity, this spice may raise blood sugar levels. After a meal, this slows the rise in blood sugar.
BERBERINE. This compound lowers blood sugar by encouraging your tissues to use sugar

and increasing insulin production while also stimulating enzymes to break down glucose.

SEEDS OF FENUGREEK There is some evidence that fenugreek may support blood sugar management, although additional high-quality studies in humans are required.

If you are already taking blood-sugar-lowering medications, you should talk to your doctor before adding any of these foods to your diet because some herbal supplements may interact negatively with them.

12. Maintain a healthy weight

Keeping a healthy weight helps maintain healthy blood sugar levels and lowers your risk of developing diabetes

Even a 5% weight loss can improve blood sugar regulation and reduce the need for diabetes medication,

For instance, if a person weighs 200 pounds (91 kilograms) and loses just 10 to 14 pounds (4.5 to 6 kilograms), their blood sugar levels may rise significantly.

Furthermore, readings of glycated hemoglobin (HbA1c) may rise if you lose more than 5% of your initial weight. These are used as indicators of your blood sugar levels over the past three months.

13. Eat healthy snacks more often

It may help you avoid both high and low blood sugar levels by spreading out your meals and snacks throughout the day.

Snacking between meals may also lower your risk of type 2 diabetes.

In fact, several studies suggest that eating smaller, more frequent meals throughout the day may increase insulin sensitivity and lower blood sugar levels.

14. Eat foods high in probiotics

Probiotics are friendly bacteria that have many health benefits, including better control of blood sugar.

Consuming probiotics may reduce insulin resistance and fasting blood sugar in people with type 2 diabetes.

Intriguingly, studies have shown that people who consume multiple species of probiotics for at least eight weeks experience greater improvements in blood sugar levels.

Fermented foods like these are probiotic-rich:

Yogurt, as long as it says on the label that it contains live and active cultures, such as kefir, tempeh, sauerkraut, or kimchi

Conclusion

Natural methods for controlling blood sugar levels abound.

Changing your lifestyle, such as managing your weight, stress levels, and quality of sleep, exercising, and drinking enough water are many of them. Nevertheless, the choices you make regarding your diet account for some of the greatest improvements.

Before changing your lifestyle or trying new supplements, check with your doctor, especially if you have trouble controlling your blood sugar or take medication.

Foods provide the body with additional benefits, including boosting immunity, repairing damaged cells, and detecting most lifestyle diseases, in addition to lowering blood sugar quickly. However, this is by no means an exhaustive list of foods that can be consumed to maintain blood sugar levels in check. This list is meant to show you some locally available foods with a low glycemic index that can be used to control blood sugar levels. In addition to consuming a healthy diet, individuals with extremely high blood sugar levels should consult a dietitian, clinical nutritionist, or their family doctor for the best treatment strategy.

www.ingramcontent.com/pod-product-compliance
Lightning Source LLC
Chambersburg PA
CBHW071137220526
45467CB00015B/1360